D1432820

You Don't Have To Live With It!™

*Uncovering nature's power
with SottoPelle®
bio-identical hormones*

By Gino Tutera, M.D., F.A.C.O.G.

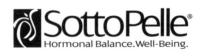

YOU DON'T HAVE TO LIVE WITH IT!©
Copyright © 2003 by Gino Tutera, M.D., F.A.C.O.G.
All rights reserved. Printed in the United States of America. No part of this book may
be used or reproduced in any manner without permission. For information, contact:
SottoPelle®, 8412 E. Shea Blvd., Suite 101, Scottsdale, AZ 85260

www.sottopelletherapy.com
Published by SottoPelle Marketing Group
5410 N. Scottsdale Rd., Suite B 200
Paradise Valley, AZ 85253
carolann@sphrt.com
480.874.1515

Library of Congress Cataloguing-in-Publication Data2003093811
ISBN: 0-9742223-0-5
First Edition: June 2003
Second Edition: November 2004
Third Edition: January 2009

TABLE OF CONTENTS

FOREWORD

Dr. Gino Tutera has more than 30 years of experience and more than a decade of documented research proving SottoPelle® is far superior to synthetic or other bio-identical hormones on the market.

Dr. Tutera successfully operates SottoPelle® centers for hormonal balance and well-being throughout Arizona and Southern California.

SottoPelle® Society is a national network of physicians who have adopted and implemented Dr. Gino Tutera's SottoPelle® Therapy for bio-identical hormone replacement and who are dedicated to health and well-being.

SottoPelle® patients want:
- To be more vital and feel younger
- Look and feel better
- Caring and compassionate medical care
- A safe and effective alternative to synthetic or other HRT
- A simple, worry-free choice. No pills to take or creams to apply
- To know they are receiving the right dosage of hormones for their body to stay at premium levels at all times
- Peace of mind

To locate a physician trained in SottoPelle® Therapy, visit Dr. Tutera's website at sottopelletherapy.com or call 480.874.1515.

ACKNOWLEDGEMENTS

To my loving wife Carolann, thank you so much for all your help and encouragement. Without you this book would never have been completed. To my son Adam, thank you for your love.

Introduction
You Really Don't!

YOU DON'T HAVE TO LIVE WITH IT! is much more than a catchy title, it is my whole purpose for continuing to practice medicine. Having to live with symptoms related to hormonal problems associated with aging, surgery, and related deficiencies is not the way it has to be either for you as a patient or for me as a physician. Consequently, I have written this book for four reasons:

1. To eliminate the statement, "You'll just have to live with it" from the vocabulary of hormone replacement therapy.

2. To help patients understand the realities of how hormones impact their bodies' daily functions.

3. To help physicians free their thinking from traditional and out-dated treatments.

4. To present a proven, well-researched therapy which has produced remarkable results for more than 1,000 of my own patients over the last ten years and has been documented or researched in medical journals since 1935 and is used in England, Australia and other countries daily.

In light of the recently discontinued national study (Women's Health Initiative) on hormone replacement therapy (HRT), the media coverage and public reactions have been extreme, to say the least. The fear and frustration this whole issue has created has left nearly everyone unsure what to do next. This is true for physicians as well as patients.

The stoppage of the study called the Women's Health Initiative (W.H.I.) due to increasing rates of breast cancer, and cardiovascular disease, caused shock waves in our society. This study demonstrated that oral conjugated estrogen, estrogen removed from horse urine, such as Premarin, especially when coupled with synthetic progesterone (i.e: Premarin™, Provera™, Prempro™, Premphase™) caused a slight increase in the rate of breast cancer cases developing in the study group. The problem with this study in the conclusion reached was that <u>all estrogen</u> caused the same problems. *This is simply illogical.* Oral conjugated estrogen (Premarin™, etc) is horse estrogen and is as different from human estrogen as night is to day. The logic that oral estrogen (Premarin™) causes an increase in breast cancer therefore all estrogen does the same is hogwash. This would be comparable to saying that because one cosmetic company produces a bad mascara that all mascaras are bad for you. This is not logical. All estrogen is not the same. The estrogen therapy promoted in this book is bio-identical, which means it is identical to that which the human body produces, and does not cause any of the problems that horse or synthetic estrogen may cause.

The hormone therapy that I use in my practice has been used in the United States since 1939, yet has been ignored because of the political agenda of pharmaceutical companies in the United States. Pellet bio-identical hormone therapy that you will learn about has had continual positive research papers published in respected international medical journals since 1935 to the present day, as seen in the bibliography. It's now time for the men and women of the United States to be offered the safety of bio-identical HRT.

Consequently, it seemed appropriate to make my insights, experiences, and expertise known to both patients and physicians. In my over 30 years of medical practice, I have seen, read, and heard many opinions on hormonal therapy for menopause, andropause (male menopause), and PMS. This issue has become extremely confusing, especially for the general public. Frankly, I hope to eliminate the confusion and shine some light on a clearer path to hormonal balance and general well-being.

Even though I am an OB/GYN physician, I have studied and maintain a keen interest in endocrinology. When I was a resident, I initiated and completed a detailed research paper on the insulin levels in the amniotic fluid of pregnant women who were diabetic. The paper was published in 1973. During the course of research, I fully acquainted myself with the human endocrine system and have since paid close attention to all the new developments in this field.

Exacerbating this confusion is the "traditional" training and thinking still prevalent in medicine today. For doctors, there isn't sufficient emphasis given on how to properly diagnose and formulate a therapy program for the hormonal problems associated with menopause and andropause. Menopause is defined as the point in time that a woman ceases ovulation and/or menstrual periods. This can be the result of normal aging or, oftentimes, in the case of younger women, becomes an issue due to surgery and the removal of the ovaries. Andropause is defined as male menopause characterized by falling testosterone levels. Additionally, virtually no physician-teaching programs mention natural hormone therapy at all. Natural hormone replacement therapy is viewed as something created by "shamans" or "voodoo" practitioners. I am convinced that this type of thinking is outdated, unrealistic and ineffective.

If you are a woman or a man seeking an end to your fears about and frustrations with hormone replacement therapy, I trust that this book will assist you in your search for a physician who will meet your needs. If you are a physician who is tired of going through the routine without fulfilling results, I invite you to read this book carefully and contact me for any additional data or research information you would like to review.

I have purposely written this book to be just a little biased on the technical side. It isn't an attempt to prove my expertise. It is, however, what I believe patients today should know about what goes on in their bodies and how the medical community looks for answers. *It is my hope that you, as a reader, will understand more clearly that the issue of hormones is complex but it need not be a deep, dark secret reserved for an elite few to understand.* This does not mean that after reading this book you will be equipped to diagnose yourself. It does mean that you will be able to ask more direct questions and seek more complete and satisfying answers from your physician.

If you are a physician who is reading this book, I want you to know that I possess scores of articles from very highly credentialed (mostly British) institutions that have been studying and recommending bio-identical hormones for decades. If you desire to research this further, please feel free to contact me for more information.

This book has been divided into eight sections following this Introduction. The summary shown below will provide the overarching purpose for each:

• **Chapter 1—Make it go away!** A look into the various symptoms associated with hormone imbalances.

• **Chapter 2—I had no idea!** A description of the various organs, their functions, their roles, and the hormones they produce and regulate.

• **Chapter 3— No wonder nothing's worked before!** A list of the laboratory tests that accurately gauge your body's proper balance.

• **Chapter 4—Been there, done that!** An analysis of some of the more common side-effect-laden treatments traditionally prescribed.

• **Chapter 5—That's what I've been looking for!** An introduction to the best therapy available today.

• **Chapter 6—Can SottoPelle® help with these?** A look at some of the more serious health issues which SottoPelle® can help alleviate.

• **Chapter 7—I feel alive again!** A portrait of what your new life will be like.

• **Conclusion—I'm ready to begin!** Where to start in your search to find someone to help you with SottoPelle® Therapy treatments.

I trust that everyone who reads this book will be helped and certainly will come to the very clear understanding that "having to live with it" is not true. There is hope, and there is a better way to feel vigorous, vital, and rejuvenated, through **SottoPelle® Therapy.**

Chapter 1
Make it go away!

All too often I have heard both my male and female patients say, "I wish this would just go away." It is an amazing fact that men and women who suffer from hormonal difficulties have the same symptoms and complaints. I have listed a full set of symptoms and problems below. These symptoms are due to estrogen and testosterone deficiencies for both sexes.

WOMEN	MEN
anxiety	anxiety
irritability	irritability
fatigue	fatigue
loss of energy	loss of energy
poor focus	poor focus
poor concentration	poor concentration
depression	depression

loss of muscle tone	loss of muscle tone
decreased exercise tolerance	decreased exercise tolerance
prolonged recovery from exercise	prolonged recovery from exercise
no improvement with exercise	no improvement with exercise
weight gain in spite of exercise	weight gain in spite of exercise
loss of memory	loss of memory
osteoporosis	osteoporosis
decreased sexual desire	decreased sexual desire
loss of cardiac	loss of cardiac
protection	protection
higher bad cholesterol	higher bad cholesterol
hot flashes	decreased erectile function
night sweats	prostate enlargement

With all the negative effects caused by estrogen and testosterone deficiency, wouldn't you want to make them just go away? Unfortunately, these problems don't take care of themselves. *Unless you take action and seek help, your overall well-being will continue to worsen.* I know there are people who say they don't have any of these problems, or that their problems "went away" by themselves. Yes, they may have had a decrease in the frequency of their symptoms, but the more serious problems of heart attack, stroke, osteoporosis, depression, and loss of mental acuity all continue to worsen. Denial is a handy method we use all too often. *We want to fix our problems ourselves but there are issues that can only be safely treated through the use of bio-identical hormones.*

Before we take a look at what to do to make these symptoms go away, it is crucial that we first examine just how complex our bodies' hormonal processes are, as well as how hormones are made and how they work.

Chapter 2
I had no idea!

Our bodies have been created to function in an environment of balanced hormones. When the body is balanced, health and well-being exist. Physical and emotional health are intimately dependent on the body being balanced physically, spiritually, emotionally and mentally.

Certain hormones are produced by a group of glands and organs in the body called the endocrine system. The endocrine glands are specialized glands that secrete their hormones directly into the blood stream. These glands and organs include the pituitary, thyroid, pancreas, adrenals, ovaries and testicles. All other glands, salivary, breast, etc. deliver their products by a tube called a duct. Ensuring that the hormones are properly delivered—at the right times and in the right amounts—into the bloodstream is the ultimate goal.

What we need to discuss first is what each endocrine gland and organ does and the function of the hormones these glands and organs produce and regulate.

THE PITUITARY (THE BODY'S CEO)

The pituitary is a bean-sized gland that sits at the base of the brain just above the area where the nerves from the eyes meet. The pituitary gland is the command center for the hormone regulation from the endocrine glands. The endocrine glands are a set of glands that secrete their hormones directly into the bloodstream and not through a tube like the glands that make sweat or saliva.

The pituitary gland is divided into two parts that sit one behind the other. The front half of the gland is called the anterior pituitary. The front half (anterior) regulates the production and release of hormones from the thyroid gland, the adrenal gland, the ovary, and the testicle. Each of these glands will be discussed individually at a later time. The back half of the pituitary gland is called the posterior pituitary. This part of the gland secretes certain hormones that only are seen in pregnancy and breastfeeding.

The pituitary gland is an endocrine gland, which means it secretes the hormones it produces directly into the bloodstream. The front half of the gland (anterior pituitary) secretes the following hormones that control and regulate the release of hormones from all the other endocrine glands except one:, the pancreas.

1. Follicle stimulating hormone (FSH)

   - controls the ovary and the testicles

2. Luteinizing hormone (LH)

   - controls the ovary and the testicles

3. Thyroid stimulating hormone (TSH)

   - controls the thyroid gland

4. Adrenocorticotropic hormone (ACTH)

   - controls the adrenal gland

In order to understand how the endocrine hormones are controlled, its important to know how the release of these hormones are regulated by the pituitary gland. The regulation process is called the "Feedback System." This "system" is a very specific but delicate process. Hopefully I can give you an understandable explanation.

Figure one is a graphic design that shows the pituitary gland, and how it works as the body's command center through a process called the "feedback system." The other glands send their hormones through the blood stream. In the pituitary gland there are specific areas which control each gland. This means that each gland has a

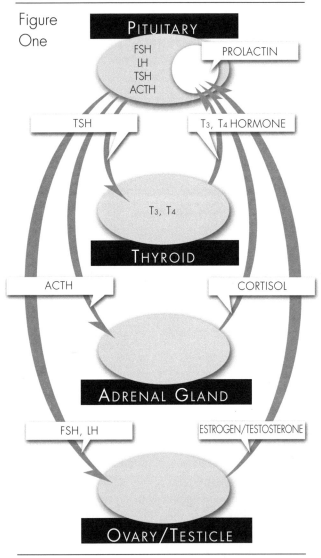

very specific site that controls a specific gland's hormone production and release, just as a bank has a loan department and a trust department. An example of how this works is as follows: (please refer back to Fig. 1) the pituitary gland through its blood supply, samples each hormone (estrogen, thyroid, etc.) in the specific area from which it is controlled. Let's take the thyroid gland as an example.

Thyroid hormone is brought to the pituitary gland and its level is determined in the thyroid area of the pituitary gland. If the thyroid gland isn't making enough hormone, the pituitary gland determines how low the level of hormone is, then releases the proper amount of the regulatory hormone, thyroid stimulating hormone, more commonly known as: TSH. (See Fig. 1). The TSH goes to the thyroid gland and tells the gland "make more hormone." The thyroid gland then makes more hormone, and as the thyroid hormone levels rise the pituitary recognizes this information and begins to decrease the release of the regulatory hormone, in this case TSH. To simply describe this <u>feedback system</u>, the pituitary gland finds a low hormone level and sends a messenger to that specific gland telling it to make more hormone. As the hormone levels rise their information "feeds back" to the pituitary gland. The level of hormone in the blood is the information that feeds back to the pituitary, which then decides if the gland is overproducing, or under producing hormone. This process is called the "feedback system" or "feedback mechanism." This process occurs rapidly. In the time it took to read the prior sentence, this process of "feed back" has taken place hundreds of times. This process continues every minute, twenty-four hours a day. The reason for this is the body needs steady levels of all hormone in the bloodstream at all times. The human body functions optimally when the levels of all hormones are kept in a steady level flow. The only method to deliver estrogen and testosterone in this steady manner for a prolonged period of time (4-6) months is with the use of SottoPelle® bio-identical hormone therapy. The description of these pellets is what this book is about.

Each of the regulatory hormones from the pituitary gland is gland specific. FSH (Follicle Stimulating Hormone) exerts its regulation on the ovary and testicles to regulate estrogen production in women and testosterone in men. LH or Leutenizing Hormone regulates the production of progesterone. TSH (Thyroid Stimulating Hormone) regulates the secretion of the thyroid hormones from the thyroid gland. ACTH regulates the secretion of cortisol from the outer shell of each adrenal gland called the cortex. Prolactin is the hormone from the posterior pituitary that is usually only secreted during pregnancy and when a woman is breast-feeding. (If prolactin is secreted in any significant amount other than in pregnancy or breast-feeding, a disease or adverse reaction to medication is present. High prolactin can stop ovulation and estrogen production. One sign of an elevated prolactin is milk production from the nipple outside of pregnancy or breast-feeding).

Clearly, you can see that if the pituitary is malfunctioning, then a considerable number of the endocrine organs can be affected. Pituitary tumors, cancerous and non-cancerous, can wreak havoc in the human body. Diseases such as Sheehan's Syndrome, which occur after the blood supply to the pituitary is stopped or suddenly reduced after delivery of a baby, can destroy the ability of the pituitary to produce regulatory hormones. This produces serious health problems.

That is why I continue to be amazed (and quite perturbed) that so many physicians who do hormone replacement for men and women, remain so hesitant to obtain blood levels of these regulatory hormones during routine evaluations or at a patient's request.

The Thyroid

The thyroid gland is found in the neck just below the "Adam's Apple." The gland is soft and spongy and usually too small to be felt. The thyroid gland helps us in various ways, but mainly it helps maintain our metabolic rate. The metabolic rate is what helps us with weight management and regulation of our body fat. This gland is controlled by the pituitary gland through a messenger hormone called the Thyroid Stimulating Hormone (TSH). TSH is the hormone that controls the thyroid glands production and release of the two thyroid hormones. These two hormones are designated T3 and T4. The underproduction of thyroid hormone is called: Hypothyroid which causes weight gain, heart trouble, intolerance for cold, and muscle weakness. If too much thyroid hormone is produced a person is said to be hyperthyroid. Excess production of the thyroid hormones or hyperthyroidism can result in marked weight changes, heart palpitations, osteoporosis (bone loss), heat intolerance and even death.

The serious consequences that can occur when the thyroid gland is improperly regulated makes it all the more important that the laboratory tests that tell us if the thyroid is working normally be interpreted properly. Later in the book, an explanation of what tests need to be done and how to properly interpret them will be given (Chapter 3).

THE ADRENAL GLANDS

The Adrenal glands are two glands that work together. They sit like hats above each kidney. Even though you have an adrenal gland on each side of the body they work as one gland. The adrenal glands have an outer covering like the peel of an orange called the cortex. This peel-like layer produces cortisone. Cortisone is very important in the way our bodies fight inflammation and infection. The production and the release of our internally manufactured cortisone (called cortisol) is regulated by the pituitary hormone ACTH. This is controlled by another feedback system. (See Fig. I). The pituitary gland sends the messenger hormone, ACTH, which tells the adrenal glands, "I'm under stress!" "Make me some cortisone" and the adrenal glands respond by making and releasing cortisone. When enough hormone is sent back to the pituitary gland through the bloodstream, the area in the pituitary that produces the messenger hormone ACTH recognizes the body has enough of the hormone cortisol and turns off the production of ACTH when enough hormone has been made. When diseases or tumors affect the adrenal glands, life-threatening conditions arise. Diseases that affect or destroy the adrenal glands can adversely affect our immune system, blood pressure, heart function, weight control and muscles.

The spongy middle of the adrenal gland, which can be compared to the pulp of an orange, is called the medulla. This spongy middle produces <u>adrenaline.</u> Adrenaline is what speeds up our heart rate, increases our blood pressure, and gets us ready to deal with stress. When we humans are under stress and we get sweaty and our hearts race, it is because of the amount of adrenaline the adrenal gland makes. The more adrenaline released, the more our heart races and the more we feel sweaty. If you ever get a shot of adrenaline to treat the effects of an allergy reaction or an attack of asthma you rapidly find out your heart speeds up significantly, making you shake, tremble and sweat.

The adrenal glands can also produce small amounts of estrogen and testosterone which can be overproduced in times of stress, or in response to disease or tumors. It is not unusual for women to develop irregular periods, acne, and fluid reten-tion as a result of stress or disease causing the adrenal glands to overproduce estrogen, testoster-one and weaker forms of male-like hormones.

The Pancreas

Blood sugar regulation and production of digestive enzymes are the main function of the pancreas. The pancreas sits to the right of the stomach, close to the gall bladder. This proximity of the gland to the gall bladder is why diseases of the gall bladder can cause the pancreas to become inflamed. The pancreas is a soft gland that has small groups of cells called the Islets of Langerhans that produce the hormone insulin. Insulin secretion is regulated by the "feedback" of the body's blood sugar to these groups of cells. When blood sugar rises, these cells produce insulin to drive the sugar into the body's cells to be utilized as fuel. When the body can no longer produce adequate insulin, the disease diabetes develops. The severity of the disease depends on how much insulin the body can produce. The less insulin produced in response to an increase in blood sugar, the more severe the disease becomes. The development of better drugs to help sufferers of this disease who still have the ability to produce some insulin has been a great step forward. These individuals usually have developed the disease as adults (Adult Onset Diabetes). The more serious form of the disease is called Insulin Dependent Diabetes. These are the individuals who must daily give themselves multiple injections of insulin to regulate their blood sugar. Researchers have determined that regulation of the body's blood sugar is best achieved with multiple doses of insulin. Research and development in insulin therapy is being undertaken to create a steady secretion of insulin that is a re-creation of what the body normally produces. Another important development is the creation of human insulin. Its use with diabetics has eliminated adverse allergies typically associated with the reactions to pig and horse insulin used in the past.

I hope that by now you are beginning to see a common thread developing through this discussion, not only related to the pancreas but to hormones overall. That thread is that bio-identical—precisely what the body produces for itself—is the secret ingredient in medicine. Side effects are diminished or eliminated when a therapy, prescribed by doctors, uses precisely the same thing naturally produced by the body to supplement the body's own functions versus a process of imitation.

The Ovaries

The two ovaries, one on each side of a woman's body, next to the uterus, have cells that produce estrogen, progesterone and testosterone. The production and release of these hormones is controlled by a feedback mechanism involving the pituitary gland's production of

<u>Follicle Stimulating Hormone</u> (FSH) and <u>Luteinizing Hormone</u> (LH). These two hormones control the production and release of estrogen and progesterone during a menstrual cycle. (See Fig. I). The pituitary hormone FSH & LH also control the process of ovulation (egg development and release). The ovaries also have certain cells that produce only testosterone. With the tremendous impact on women of estrogen, progesterone, and testosterone deficiency, a separate chapter will be devoted to this alone including treatment with the ultimate bio-identical hormone replacement: <u>SottoPelle® Therapy</u>.

The Testicles

In men the testicles are responsible for testosterone hormone production and sperm production as well. Like the ovary, the testicles are controlled by the pituitary gland's production of FSH and LH through the feedback mechanism. (See Fig. I). Unlike the ovary, the testicle only produces one hormone, testosterone, when functioning normally. Men can produce small amounts of estrogen but it's not made by any cell in the testicle but rather by the transformation of testosterone into the hormone estrogen by an enzyme. How this all happens will be further explained in subsequent chapters.

Hormones. We all need them!

Human hormones are substances our bodies produce to regulate and stimulate many organ systems. Without normal levels of hormones, our bodies are swept into a state of chaos and disease. Hormones keep us on a normal balanced path which helps us maintain our "wellness" rather than be affected with an "illness." *Often physicians forget how important proper hormone balance is to the maintenance of overall well-being. This often leads to patients not being evaluated completely and being told or made to feel that what they are experiencing is "all in your head." In truth, many of the feelings of illness can be hormone-based and the imbalance of their hormones is not imaginary.*

The previous discussion on control of hormone production and release, ie: "feedback system," (see Fig. I), I hope has been sufficient to give you at least a superficial understanding how the pituitary, thyroid, pancreas, adrenals, ovaries and testicles (the endocrine glands) work. We now should look to how hormones are made.

The thyroid gland makes thyroid hormone from iodine. The body sends iodine to the thyroid where the iodine is made into the two thyroid hormones T3 and T4. Under the control of the pituitary, the thyroid will slow down or speed up the production of the thyroid hormones through the actions of TSH. TSH (thyroid stimulating hormone) is, as we discussed, produced in a specific area of the pituitary gland) our body's CEO). When enough thyroid hormone is in the blood, the pituitary turns off the TSH and the thyroid stops its production of thyroid hormone. If the thyroid can no longer produce enough hormone for the body, treatment is necessary. Natural thyroid is what I would advise using and certainly patients have the absolute right to ask his or her physician to prescribe that particular hormone. Remember the best way to treat a hormone deficiency is to use a biologically identical form of the hormone to be replaced. Sometimes surgery is needed as well if a tumor is present.

The adrenal gland production of its hormone cortisol, is governed by the pituitary gland's secretion of ACTH (see Fig. I) through a "feed-back system." The adrenal hormone presently does not have a biologically identical treatment available at this time, and the standard forms of therapy are all that can be used.

The pancreas produces an endocrine hor-mone insulin, and has its own internal control or feedback mechanism. The groups of cells that produce insulin, which keeps the blood sugar normal, are called the Islets of Langerhans. Then cells produce insulin in response to the level of sugar present in the blood. The pituitary gland doesn't function in this process. The Islets control themselves. Historically if insulin were necessary, it was obtained from pigs and horses. These forms of insulin caused significant problems with adverse reactions. This was rectified when human insulin was developed. In addition, better control of the blood sugar has been obtained by the use of multiple injections, because the blood sugar level stays much more level. In fact, this prompted the development of a machine called the insulin pump which gives a steady stream of insulin continuously. This releases biologically identical hormone in a low-dose steady stream and has the capability to give more when needed. This is the perfect model for replacing all endocrine hormones.

The last hormones to be discussed are estrogen, testosterone and progesterone. Figure two demonstrates in a simple way how our bodies make these hormones. As you can see everything starts with the cholesterol molecule. If one's diet is inadequate, it can affect your hormones output.

Human hormones are substances our bodies produce to regulate, stimulate, and affect many organ systems. Without these, many of the things we do every day would be impossible.

Figure Two

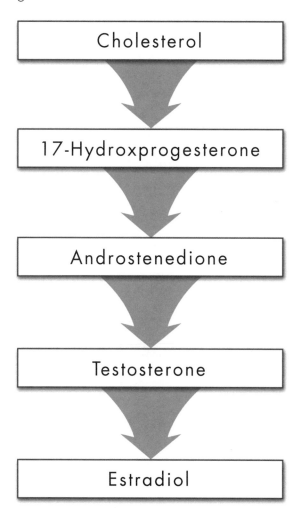

Hormones keep us on a normal, balanced path to maintain our wellness. When our bodies' natural processes are interrupted, we are placed in an unbalanced, diseased state. This means that we would find ourselves in a physical, mental, and emotional state termed "illness."

How often have you or someone you know been told, "It's all in your head?" In truth, many of the things we see or experience as feeling ill are hormone based, and the imbalance of hormones produced in our bodies caused these problems. They are not imaginary!

Estrogen from the Ovaries

The body makes three different estrogens: estrone, estradiol and estriol. The major estrogen in a woman is estradiol. In fact, it is produced in amounts twice as great as the levels of estrone in the blood. This ratio of estradiol to estrone normally is 2:1. To normally function a women's body has to have this ratio of estrogens present. If the ratio is changed, it would cause too much estrone to be made, and this estrogen is a very strong breast stimulator. One reason women complain of breast tenderness while on oral estrogens is because all oral estrogens do not keep the normal ratio of estradiol to estrone at 2:1. In fact the ratio seen with Premarin and all tablets containing conjugated estrogens is a complete reversals of this ratio to 1:2. The oral estradiol (i.e. Estrace) tablets usually make the normal ratio of 2:1 change to 1:1. This identical ratio is also seen with the estradiol used in all the estrogen patches. The only form of estrogen therapy that reproduces the normal ratio of estrogens in the body are the type used in SottoPelle® Therapy (estradiol pellets). Dr. M. Thom in her articles published in 1980 and 1981 in the British Journal of Medicine and British Journal of OB/GYN demonstrated this very elegantly.

A few comments regarding estriol. Estriol has been touted as an estrogen that does not cause breast cancer. The evidence for this is faulty. The amount of estriol used in these studies was so low that the estrogen level in the blood would be very low. If enough estriol is given to produce a relief of symptoms of the menopause such as vaginal dryness and changing of hot flashes, the dosage would be 2 to 4 times the amount used in these studies. In fact any estrogen given in doses that equal the doses used in these studies would also show no increase in the incidence of breast cancer.

This leads to only one conclusion. Give women the estrogen the body uses commonly, estradiol. Furthermore, recreate the normal ratio of estradiol to the other estrogens, 2:1. And remember, the only form of estrogen replacement therapy that can

do all of this is biologically identical SottoPelle®
Therapy and the use of estradiol pellets.

Nutritional Supplements

I know there are numerous authors touting their
supplements, but nutritional supplements can
be dangerous through overuse. Pregnenalone
and DHEA carry definite risks and should only
be used if nothing else is available, and only
in strict moderation. With the scheme of how
our bodies make estrogen and testosterone,
you need to realize that all the other substances
offered as supplements, often taken in combination, can cause physiologic harm to our bodies.
Pregnenalone and DHEA both help the body
make testosterone, but no study has been done
to establish a safe amount of either compound.
If you have a normal estrogen and testosterone
level in the blood your body doesn't need DHEA
or Pregnenalone.

Testosterone

Both men and women produce testosterone.
Figure two gives a simple diagram of how testosterone is made. Men produce over 99% of their
testosterone in certain cells of the testicle and
1% from the adrenal gland. Women produce
testosterone primarily from their ovaries and a tiny
amount from the adrenal glands.

Postmenopausal women continue to produce testosterone from their ovaries even after estrogen production has stopped.

Without the proper levels of testosterone, men and women experience loss of mental focus and concentration. The lack of testosterone also produces muscle loss, decreased strength, fatigue, poor response to exercise, loss of libido (sex drive and arousal), and worsened menopausal symptoms in women. Anxiety and irritability are increased in both men and women suffering from lack of testosterone.

If men and women suffer when they are testosterone deficient, how should this be treated? The best option is natural biologically identical testosterone. Synthetic and chemically treated testosterone can cause serious problems such as facial hair, baldness, acne, liver problems and prostate problems. Biologically identical testosterone is least likely to cause problems, especially when used in pellet form. The injection of synthetic testosterone causes the "roller coaster" effect just like estrogen injection. (The "roller coaster" effect is seen in the blood levels when bio-equivalent synthetic replicas pills, patches, or creams are used. The up and down swings of hormones are produced as a result of the length of the life cycle of each form of hormone therapy.

The shorter the life of the hormone, the faster the rise and decline of the hormone levels in the blood.) Oral forms of testosterone, unless they are bio-identical, can cause liver problems. To be complete, testosterone gels and creams are available, but they have to be applied many times daily to try and reproduce normal blood levels, which they don't. The only form of bio-identical testosterone that recreates the natural blood levels the body needs over an extended period (three to six months) is pellet therapy. To summarize, the only form of testosterone therapy that is safe and effective, is the type of bio-identical testosterone pellets used in SottoPelle® Therapy.

The last aspect to be addressed is how SottoPelle® testosterone therapy benefits men and women. Other forms of testosterone therapy have major drawbacks—patches, creams, tablets, and injections—all of which produce a pronounced roller coaster effect. Furthermore, they enhance the production of a protein called SHBG (sex hormone binding globulin) into the blood that attaches itself to testosterone and renders it useless. SottoPelle® hormones do not produce any of these negative effects. Following initiation of pellet testosterone therapy, both sexes can expect increased sexual arousal, increased libido, improved mental acuity, improved mental focus and concentration, improved muscle tone, less fatigue, more energy, and improved bone density. Testosterone is a great bone builder and lack of it leads to the development of osteoporosis. The use of SottoPelle® gives the body the doses needed over a long period of time that allows for improved bone production.

Chapter 3
No wonder nothing's worked before!

The errors in diagnosis and treatment made by physicians usually result from not getting lab work, not getting the correct lab work, or not knowing what the lab work means. Therefore you need to find a caregiver who uses a scientific approach to hormone therapy. This means someone who gets the proper lab work to make the diagnosis and, more importantly, rechecks the lab work after therapy begins to assess the success of the therapy.

So many times patients have presented themselves to me with lab work indicating normal hormone levels, but there is no measurement of the corresponding regulatory hormone. When they were re-evaluated with the appropriate tests, nearly all of them had blood work that indicated a need for hormone therapy, or it showed that their present therapy was ineffective. This is a consistently reoccurring finding in my practice.

In most cases their complaints to their caregivers go unheeded or ignored. This often causes great anxiety and depression. A patient whose lab work indicated normal levels but is unaware that the caregiver has not measured the regulatory hormone, has been done a great disservice. As patients, they have the feeling something is wrong, but when they hear that "everything is normal" and, therefore, "it's all in your head," they can't help but feel frustrated and helpless.

We physicians are not taught to check or recheck estrogen or FSH lab values. We are taught to use the "I feel okay" test. If the patient complains of feeling miserable and "feels okay" after a pill is given, then the physician is led to believe that he/she has done a "good job."

Why is this the standard? The answer is ignorance. Estrogen therapy has been practiced as if hormone pills are candy. Give a patient the green one or the red one or another yellow one until they say they are O.K. Job done! Where is the laboratory evidence before and after a hormone is given? For all other types of illnesses, doesn't a good physician thoroughly and properly check all appropriate laboratory tests before and after all other types of treatments have been administered to verify that the chosen therapy is effective? Why should the approach to hormone therapy be any different? Lab work is critical before and after any hormone therapy. Demand it! Don't be intimidated into believing you don't need lab work. It is essential!

What tests do I need?

How can so many men and women have the same complaints and yet proper investigation is not undertaken? Through proper interpretation of laboratory tests, most problems caused by hormone deficiency can be diagnosed and treated. The following discussion will help explain what tests need to be done and how to make sense of the information obtained.

Thyroid Tests

•TSH

TSH is the hormone that comes from the human pituitary gland (see Fig. I) that controls the thyroid gland. It regulates the production of the two thyroid hormones. (See Chapter 2) To review - the two thyroid hormones are called T3 and T4. The scientific names are long and difficult to remember but if you talk to a physician using the terms T3 and T4 will be enough.

Measuring TSH levels in the blood are the gold standard for finding an overactive (hyperthyroid or underactive (hypothyroid) thyroid gland.

By measuring the level of this hormone, a diagnosis of whether the thyroid gland is making a proper amount of hormone can be made. If the thyroid gland is producing enough hormone, the TSH level will be in the normal range. The normal range is usually a number between one and five in most laboratories. The thyroid gland when it produces too much hormone is said to be "overactive" or the person is said to be hyperthyroid. If this is the case the blood level of TSH will be low (below the lowest normal number for the laboratory that does the test.) The person who has an underactive thyroid has a thyroid gland that is not producing enough thyroid hormone. Such a person is termed hypothyroid. The TSH level in the blood is higher than the highest number of the normal range: ie: 5.0 or above. The higher the level of TSH, the lower the level of thyroid hormone in the blood. The diagnosis of whether the thyroid gland is overactive or underactive can only be made by accurately finding the level of TSH in the blood. If the level of the two thyroid hormones is all that is checked, an incorrect diagnosis is often made and thyroid hormone may be improperly given.

•T3 (Triodothyronine)

One of the hormones produced by the thyroid is T3. The scientific name is a tongue-twister, so

T3 will be used. The measurement of the blood level of T3 is usually reported as a measurement of the total amount of this particular thyroid hormone. The correct interpretation of laboratory test results requires the physician to recognize that certain conditions (i.e.: pregnancy) and certain drugs (i.e.: birth control pills) will affect the test. The reason these conditions and drugs affect the test is they cause the body to produce certain proteins that attach themselves to the hormone T3 and make the level look higher or lower than the true level in the blood. This makes it even more important that your physician always get a measurement of the pituitary hormone TSH so that proper interpretation of the T3 lab value can be achieved.

•T4 (Thyroxine)

T4 is the other thyroid hormone produced by the thyroid glands. The laboratory tests to determine the level of T4 in the blood have been available for a long time, but once again the correct interpretation of these values relies on having the TSH tested as well. To try and say that some one has too much or too little T4 in their blood can only be done by looking at the blood level of TSH at the same time. There are two tests to find the amount of T4 thyroid hormone: total T4 and Free T4. The total T4 measure all the T4 in the blood, and free T4 measures the entire T4 hormone in the blood that is biologically available to the body. No matter which tests a physician uses it, it must be interpreted only when the level of TSH in the blood is known.

Here are some examples of what we have just discussed:

o T3 – low, T4 – normal, TSH – normal

This situation is commonly seen with women on birth control pills, hormone replacement therapy, or who are pregnant. This is someone with normal thyroid function or Euthyroid. Unfortunately, it is not uncommon for this person to be treated with a thyroid hormone, which is completely inappropriate.

o T3 – low, T4 – low, TSH – high

This is a classic example of a person with low thyroid function. This person needs thyroid hormone. This condition is called hypothyroidism. Both thyroid hormones are low, and the TSH consequently has to be high. The pituitary is sending its messenger saying: make more hormone!

o T3 – high, T4 – high, TSH – low

This is an example of a person with an overactive thyroid. This person may need drug therapy or surgery, depending on the cause. This condition is called hyperthyroidism. Both thyroid hormones are being overproduced and with high levels of hormone the pituitary shuts down the production of its thyroid-regulating hormone TSH.

Far too many people are on natural thyroid supplements who don't need the hormone. They are at risk for arrhythmia (abnormal heart rhythm) of the heart, burning out their own thyroid, and osteoporosis if used too long. It is imperative that patients be evaluated with the appropriate tests for thyroid hormone levels (T3 and T4), and have these values compared with the level of thyroid stimulating hormone (TSH).

•Estrogen and FSH

Estrogen is produced primarily in the ovaries. In humans, three estrogens are produced. (See Fig. 3) These three are estrone (E1), estradiol (E2), and estriol (E3). Estradiol is the most important estrogen in women. Estradiol is the estrogen hormone the body needs and utilizes the most.

Estradiol is the major hormone in a woman's system; the other estrogens are made from estradiol. If a woman needs estrogen, she only needs her estradiol level evaluated because the body uses this to make any estrogen it needs.

Figure Three

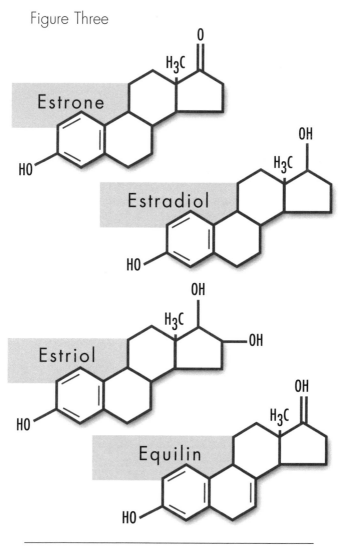

Therefore, ask only for an estradiol level to be done. More importantly, ask for your FSH, the regulatory hormone, to be measured, as well. You learn more from the FSH than any other test. Why? The FSH level gives true meaning to what a blood or saliva measurement indicates. Proper interpretation of the estrogen level in the body can only be achieved if the estradiol levels and FSH level are measured immediately and together. The reason blood tests for estrogen were given a bad reputation is the results were interpreted without a proper FSH level taken.

Samples of Lab Test Results

o Estradiol – low, FSH – high (above 23)

This patient is estrogen-deficient and needs estrogen therapy. The low estrogen hormone level causes the pituitary gland to produce high levels of FSH which is what causes the severe menopausal symptoms women experience.

o Estradiol – normal, FSH high (above 23)

This patient needs estrogen, as well, which most physicians and caregivers miss or don't understand. If they only had asked for an FSH, they wouldn't have missed the diagnosis. The FSH level being high means the body is not getting enough estrogen.

o Estradiol – normal, FSH – normal (less than 23)

This patient needs no hormonal therapy.

Testosterone (total and free) and FSH (for men and women)

Testosterone measurement is achieved by obtaining both the total and free levels of testosterone in the blood. Why both? Because the body produces a protein—Sex Hormone Binding Globulin (SHBG)—that will render testosterone ineffective in men and women. This is the reason that the total testosterone and the biologically available (free testosterone) need to be measured. The higher the SHBG activity, the lower the bio-available testosterone will be. Recent research has conclusively shown that estrogen will raise the level of SHBG in the blood and drive down the free testosterone. You need both tests to assess if testosterone therapy is appropriate and needed. Below are examples of how tests need to be interpreted.

Examples:

o Testosterone – normal; free testosterone – normal; FSH normal

No therapy needed.

o Testosterone – normal; free testosterone – low; FSH normal

Testosterone is probably needed, but this may mean that too much testosterone is being bound with sex hormone binding globulin (SHBG). The free testosterone being low indicates that there is very little testosterone available for the body to use.

o Testosterone – low; free testosterone – low

This person needs testosterone therapy.

Chapter 4
Been there, done that!
A review of common, "traditional" treatments

The use of SottoPelle® hormone replacement for men and women is far superior to any other form of administration and type available. This rather strong statement needs analysis. A look at the forms of therapy will help to show why SottoPelle® is so superior.

First, what properties would the ultimate hormone replacement possess? They would be:

- Biologically identical

- Effective and hassle-free

- Biologically available when needed 24/7

- Safe – no liver involvement

- No side effects

- Last up to six months

- No increase in breast cancer

Conjugated Estrogens

The first and most common form of estrogen utilized throughout the world (over 70%) of the market) is conjugated estrogen (Premarin, Prephase, Prempro). Conjugated estrogens are extracted from pregnant mares' urine. To use this hormone, you must accept its source. Horse estrogen is great for horses and ponies, not for humans. The chemical structure of this estrogen is completely alien to our physiologic system. Humans don't make a hormone called Equilin, (see Fig. 3) which is the prominent hormone in Premarin. This hormone changes the normal estrogen ratio in the body, which is Estradiol to Estrone from 2:1 to 1:2. This reversal causes the body to be subjected to an excess of estrone, which is a very strong breast receptor stimulant. This excess of estrone is the primary reason many women on conjugated estrogen complain of breast tenderness, water retention, and weight gain around the waist and hips. This excess could also be a factor in the increase of cases of breast cancer, after long-term usage.

To be fair, let's see if conjugated estrogen fulfills any of the properties of the ultimate hormone replacement therapy.

•Is it biologically identical? NO!

It uses equilin, a hormone made by horses, not by humans.

•Is it effective, hassle-free with no side effects? NO!

The use of conjugated estrogen does stop hot flashes, but often lab work demonstrates inadequate depression of FSH. This may explain why symptoms often reappear when stress and worry arise. As for being hassle free, you must take it every day or the effect is lost quickly.

•Is it biologically available when needed 24/7? NO!

Oftentimes, when you need hormones at the end of the day, it may not be available. (See Fig. 4, Page 56). Anything taken orally produces the roller-coaster effect of rapid rise and fall. In effect, if you need hormones late in the day, you may not have sufficient hormone for your needs—anxiety, irritability, hot flashes and insomnia may occur. This form of estrogen is not available when your body needs it.

•Is it safe? NO!

All conjugated estrogen must be processed in the liver to be activated for the body's use. This causes a rise in clotting factors which increases the chance of clots in your veins and of pulmonary embolus (clot in the lung), which can be lethal. The safety record for conjugated estrogen in relation to breast cancer has been studied and reports have indicated a 10% increase in occurrence if used over 10 years. No one should subject themselves to these risks.

The other oral synthetics (i.e.: Estrace, Menest, Estratest) also carry the same inherent properties as conjugated estrogen. The only difference is they have not been studied individually, and may potentially be more beneficial than conjugated estrogen.

Estradiol Patches

The next type of commonly used form of HRT estrogen is estradiol delivered in the form of a patch. Subjecting patch estrogen to the same test yields the following results:

•Is it biologically identical? NO!

It is synthetic estradiol, but is derived from plant sources. Pharmaceutical companies include anything made from plants as "natural." (For example, plastics are also made from plants.) Biologically identical hormones are only made by small compounding pharmacies who specialize in their production.

•Is it effective and hassle free? NO!

Patch delivered estradiol (PDE) is effective in controlling hot flashes, but its effect on bone reabsorption and prevention of heart disease is not well established. The only real difference in various patches is how long they last. For all patches, the primary problem is the adhesive. A lot of them don't stick and if they come loose, their effectiveness ends. In addition, women often complain of the irritating nature of the adhesive on the skin, and many women discontinue the patches because of adhesive problems.

•Is it biologically available when needed? NO!

The patch has a more prolonged effect than oral tablets but still has the roller coaster effect. This may lead to the development of anxiety and hot flashes when at the end of its useful life. (See Page 56).

•Is it safe? Somewhat.

The patch allows the hormone to be absorbed; therefore, it bypasses the liver for activation. You don't get the increase in clotting factors, as seen in tablets. The question regarding breast cancer in regard to patches has not been individually studied, but patches cause a more even distribution of estradiol to estrone 1:1. This is still not the natural ratio of 2:1, but it is better than Premarin.

Hormone Shots

Hormone shots of estrogen and testosterone given in the muscle are used to treat deficiencies of these hormones. Are they the answer? NO! They are synthetic—pure and simple.

•Is it biologically identical? Absolutely NOT!

No injectable biologically identical hormone is available. All shots are synthetic. No good things can be said of hormones given by injection into the muscle.

•Is it biologically available when needed? NO!

Hormones given in shot form are absorbed in a very irregular fashion that causes very irregular blood levels. This is the major reason very few doctors use shots. They are unreliable.

•Is it effective and hassle free? NO!

Initially shots are effective in making symptoms go away, but long-term use is not possible. Increased resistances to the synthetic hormones build as the shots are given. Their resistance results in patients having to get these shots more frequently. Furthermore, these injections are painful and will cause scarring in the muscle with such frequent use.

•Is it safe? NO!

Synthetic hormones are not safe in any form. Shots are the last form of therapy that should ever be used. The irregular absorption of these hormones causes blood levels of hormones to be very irregular, which causes a significant roller coaster effect. Never use injections!

Bio-identical Hormones

Recently more physicians are having biologically identical hormones made in special pharmacies called compounding pharmacies. These pharmacies hand-make custom compound hormones for patients. This has been the best development in hormone therapy. The only problem with these is that they need to be swallowed, applied in a cream from or administered in sublingual (under the tongue) tablets. Using the test questions, let's look at how they rate.

•Is it biologically identical? YES, thankfully.

•Is it effective and hassle free? NOT REALLY.

The hormones that are compounded (hand-made from individual components) and administered through capsules, creams, or sublingual tablets don't necessarily relieve the majority of patients' symptoms at low doses, as SottoPelle® hormone pellets do. Usually they have to be taken twice a day to be effective and they can be expensive, as well. In addition, the doses taken have to be high to be effective- 5–10 mg a day, which equates to 150-300 mg per month. This is a lot of hormone, but it is necessary for some women to "feel better." The use of these forms of hormones is labor intensive for patients, especially if they are using creams. The creams are messy and expensive and have a very short useful life in the body. This often leads to frequent use or under use which results in the return of all the problems. The sublingual tablets are placed under the tongue and may take a long time to dissolve if not made properly. They often need to be taken twice daily for proper hormone levels. The problem with sublingual is the compounding pharmacies must be experienced in their production or a useless tablet is produced.

•Is it biologically available when needed? NO!

These forms of therapy all produce the same roller coaster effect that all short-acting tablets, patches and cream-delivered hormones generate.

•Is it safe? YES!

Biologically identical hormone is the one form of hormone that is safe. The safety is increased if it is absorbed directly into the blood stream. In other words, don't swallow it, absorb it (cream or sublingual tablets). No increase in breast cancer has been shown thus far with the use of biologically identical hormones.

The Progesterone Myth

Progesterone is an important hormone but it's been given almost mythical status. If you believe John Lee, M.D., it can resolve the majority of perimenopausal and menopausal problems women face. He and others tout natural progesterone as a bone builder and a perfect alternative to estrogen. This is only partially correct. The use of progesterone cream has expanded dramatically in the U.S. since he published his book (What Your Doctor May Not Tell You About Menopause, May 1996). In the rest of the world, where pellet hormones are commonly used, the application of natural progesterone cream is infrequent or is completely ignored. Why the disparity? Why do physicians in other countries prefer to use natural estradiol and testosterone rather than natural progesterone? Research done throughout the world does not support progesterone as the "wonder hormone."

For women and men, progesterone production occurs as a transitional stage on the way to making estradiol and testosterone. (See Fig. 2). This simple diagram shows exactly what the body does with progesterone. Progesterone does not perpetually reside in the body nor does it have all the effects the public is led to believe. In fact, progesterone is only produced in substantial amounts in a non-pregnant woman's body for ten days of each month, and daily production of progesterone is seen only during pregnancy. Women who breast-feed do not produce progesterone and do well.

The research quoted in all the books is based on research done with synthetic progesterone, not natural progesterone. Frankly, the research done using natural progesterone has been very disappointing. One example is a study performed at UCLA medical school, and presented at the Anti Aging Association of America in Las Vegas, Nevada, based on Dr. Leonetti's work. It was conclusively demonstrated that progesterone cream at ten times the strength of the creams recommended by John Lee, M.D., and others, (which is twice the prescription strength normally ordered), produced no bone growth after a year's usage by a large study group of women. Obviously, progesterone cream is no wonder treatment. It is also not nearly as effective as it is publicized to be protecting against heart attack, stroke, Alzheimer's, and osteoporosis.

Chapter 5
That's what I've been looking for!

History of Bio-Identical Hormones

I n 1935 the insertion of estrogen and testosterone in the form of pellets began in Europe. This form of therapy was created to supply hormones to young women who had undergone a hysterectomy. This became a very successful form of estrogen and testosterone therapy. It was then given to women who had not undergone a hysterectomy with excellent results as long as progesterone was also given.

Based upon all the data and discussion in the previous chapters, man-made, bio-equivalent hormones which have to be either swallowed, injected, or topically applied are not consistently effective, are burdened with many negative side effects, and do not provide consistent, evenly distributed hormones. The best form of hormone replacement is one that is biologically identical, is directly absorbable into the bloodstream, and gives you hormones when you need them just as the ovaries and testes do. With more than a decade of research and over 26 years of experience, SottoPelle® Therapy is far superior than other forms of bio-identical HRT on the market.

Let's make sure that we clearly understand the difference between bio-equivalent and bio-identical. Bio-identical means biologically identical to what the human body produces. The definition of natural (compared to what pharmaceutical companies use) is a hormone made from a plant source. In order for a hormone to be truly natural, it needs to have the precise, biologically-identical chemical structure of the human hormone, not simply a laboratory-created chemical equivalent, which is what synthetic hormones (like Premarin™, Estrace™, Cenestin™, Estratest™, and Menest™ are). Human bodies need and want biologically-identical hormones to replace what they have lost or are unable to produce. The replacement or augmenting of hormones lost by aging or surgery must be with bio-identical hormones to ensure that the previously mentioned problems do, in fact, "go away."

In 1935, hormone pellet insertion for menopausal women was created. In 1939 Robert Greenblatt, M.D. introduced this therapy to North America. SottoPelle® Therapy, using bio-identical hormone pellets, consists of placing tiny estradiol and testosterone pellets painlessly under the skin in the fatty tissue. These pellets are similar to the size of a grain of rice. The effects of each implantation can last from four to six months or even longer. The hormone levels achieved by SottoPelle® Therapy are the closest thing to natural hormone levels produced by the human ovary and testes. (See Fig. 4) The hormone levels achieved are constant, steady, and predictable. **No other form of hormone delivery can produce a consistent blood level of estradiol and testosterone.**

Hormone pills, whether natural or synthetic, produce a "roller coaster" effect. (See Fig. 4) The pills give high levels of hormones two to four hours after ingesting them and the levels decrease steadily after that. In some individuals, their hormone levels may be so low 12 hours later that they need to take another dose but are not permitted to do so by prescription limitations. Once-daily pills are absolutely the furthest thing from the natural rhythm of hormonal secretion. The ovary and testes are designed to secrete hormones 24 hours a day. SottoPelle® Therapy, in the form of hormone pellets, is the only one that recreates the body's natural hormone-producing rhythm. The use of pills and patches can never recreate the hormone levels given through pellet therapy. More importantly, pills or patches

Figure Four

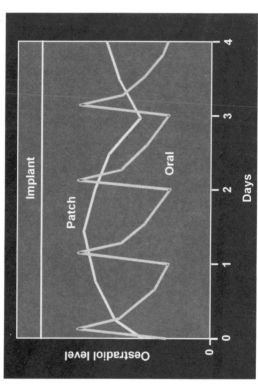

E2 Level Pills, Patches vs. Pellets

Smith, R./Studd, J.W.W.
Brit Jour Hosp Med, 1993, Vol 49, No 11

cannot respond with increased dosages of hormones when the body asks for more hormones. In contrast, SottoPelle® is always available for the body to take what it wants when it wants it, no matter what amount is needed. This property alone sets SottoPelle® Therapy far ahead of pill or patch usage in recreating a balanced hormonal environment.

The reasons hormonal deficiency in estrogen and testosterone are so well corrected by SottoPelle® Therapy using estradiol and testosterone pellets are: 1) normal levels of each hormone are achieved in the blood utilizing very low dosages of each hormone; 2) SottoPelle® Therapy releases hormones directly into the blood stream, thereby bypassing the liver; 3) SottoPelle® Therapy is the only form of hormone therapy that can release more hormone when the body demands it; and 4) SottoPelle® Therapy is made of pure crystallized, biologically identical estradiol and testosterone.

So if this therapy is so superior, why isn't it widely utilized in the United States? The primary reason is lack of exposure through marketing and advertising. A further reason pellets have not been widely utilized is the simple economic fact that the formula cannot be patented. This means that pharmaceutical companies cannot monopolize a market and, therefore, cannot generate significant profits. Consequently, the machinery of marketing and physician-training has been kept relatively small.

"Implants bypass the intestine, avoiding the first-pass effect on liver metabolism of the hormone. This prevents the unphysiological ratio of oestradiol [estradiol] to oesterone [esterone] found with oral preparations" (Thom, M, Studd, J., Oestorgen/testosterone implant therapy. Oestrogens and the Menopause 1978).

"Oral estrogen results in minor increase in clotting studies – consistent with recent studies showing no improvement in heart attack and stroke, because of their "First Pass" through the liver" Smith, RNJ, Studd, J.W.W. British Journal of Hospital Medicine 1993

"Oral preparations, unlike implants, also reduce liver metabolism of clotting factors and lipids" Elkik F., Gompel A., MTP Press 103-25

Let's look at SottoPelle® Therapy in relation to the use of synthetic hormones and also the way hormones are administered.

Estradiol and testosterone levels in the human body need to exist in sufficient quantities to satisfy the body's needs. The question is, how much hormone needs to be given to achieve normal (physiologic) levels of each hormone? If you try to achieve normal human levels with pills, a significant amount of hormone must be given. For example, the smallest dose of oral estrogen hormone available is 0.3 mg (Premarin). This means that you take in a minimum of 9.75 mg of estrogen hormone monthly (30 days times 0.3mgm). Estrace at 0.5mg daily gives you 15mgm monthly. Compare this to the estradiol given in SottoPelle® Therapy, which results in giving only 0.5 mg to 3 mg monthly. Only estradiol patches at a dosage of 0.025 mg, can deliver such low amounts of estrogen as do pellets. Why do pills have to be given in such high doses? The reason is that hormones given orally have to be processed in the liver to be activated. This process is termed "first pass metabolism." "First pass" is the passage of a substance through the liver cells in order to activate or deactivate the substance. This requires activation of an enzyme system in the body of the cell. The substances are released into the blood stream along with their byproducts. This causes stimulation of other substances in the liver to be produced such as clotting factors. These substances can have a damaging effect on the liver cells themselves causing scarring and possibly a loss of liver function. The oral hormone has to be given in such high doses to compensate for the predictable loss of hormone in the liver, and the loss of usable hormone in the intestinal tract from lack of absorption. Consequently, high doses need to be given so that only a fraction of the hormone taken in by the body ever finds its way into the bloodstream and is available for supplying the body's hormonal needs. The rest remains in the liver or is lost in the stool.

The high doses of estrogen produce the unwanted effects of breast tenderness, over-stimulation of the estrogen receptors of the breast tissue, and significant weight gain and fat deposits. The high doses of estrogen destroy the natural distribution ratios of estrogen in the blood. This also adds to the unwanted side effects produced by oral hormones. The question that has to be asked is, why swallow a hormone when the body prefers to absorb it? The producers of these oral synthetic hormones have no real answers.

Pellets are produced by pharmacies and pharmaceutical companies in Europe and many other nations. Why are they suppressed here? It seems that it's all about profits. Why would a person use anything else if the general public were as well-informed about pellets as they are about oral synthetic hormones?

As you can now see, the method of absorption profoundly influences the effect of estradiol and testosterone in the human body. Why then shouldn't these hormones be given in a way that is nearly identical to the way the body releases hormones into the blood stream? Remember that the hormone FSH regulates the flow of estrogen in the body. The human body desires the steadiest and most consistent hormonal level possible even when confronted with physical or emotional stress. The human body regulates the levels of all secreted hormones to deal with these changes, both external and internal, that affect the secretion of hormones in the human body. The only form of hormone delivery that can recreate what the body does naturally is a hormone delivery system such as SottoPelle® Therapy.

The type of hormone pellet used in SottoPelle® Therapy, be it estradiol or testosterone, is a tiny, solid cylinder (approx. 3mm in diameter) about the size of a small grain of rice. The skin is first prepared by numbing it with a small amount of Novocaine, similar to the numbing effect you receive from the dentist. The pellets are placed under the skin, with the use of a needle instrument placed into the fatty tissue. The entire procedure takes less than a few minutes. Best of all, the procedure is completely pain free.

The outer surface of this cylinder is the active area of hormone delivery. A small percentage of each pellet's surface area is released on a daily basis over a twenty-four hour period. This steady secretion keeps the level of hormones consistent in the blood stream. But what happens if you exert significant physical demands upon your body, such as exercise? Or what occurs when you experience or emotional stress, like a surprise visit from your supervisor or in-laws? If you are taking oral hormones or are wearing a patch, you will most probably be left without the appropriate hormonal reserves because pills, patches and shots cannot give you the hormones required immediately. Estradiol and testosterone pellets, like the type used in SottoPelle® Therapy, can do this because the increase in heart rate and muscle activity will generate a faster release of hormone from the surface area of the pellet, thereby releasing more hormones. When the stress ends, the body returns to its normal heart rates and activity and the release of hormones returns to its usual level.

SottoPelle® Therapy is the only option which enables your body to access hormones when it needs them. More importantly, this can be reproduced many times throughout the day and no oral tablets, shots or creams can do this. The hormone patches cannot respond quickly or sufficiently enough to satisfy the body's needs. What the human body needs to correct a hormone deficiency is the biologically identical hormone it lacks. This is common sense. Doesn't it seem right that the human body would prefer using an identical hormone? Of course it would. Synthetic hormones (bio-equivalent), whether made from plants or animal products, are just reasonable facsimiles.

"Testosterone pellet implants have many of the ideal features of a long-acting androgen depot [storage], including being safe, highly effective with stable clinical and biochemical effects, economical, providing flexible dosing, and excellent long-acting properties due to a near-zero-order dissolution. A single biodegradable implant of 600-1200 mg provides stable, effective, and well-tolerated replacement for 4-6 months and pellets can provide excellent androgen replacement in most physiological settings" (David J. Handelsman, Pharmacology, Biology, and Clinical Applications of Androgen, 1994).

Putting this all together, if a person is deficient in estradiol or testosterone, replacing that hormone with the bio-identical hormone it needs, given in the identical secretion pattern, seems the logical choice. To further bolster this statement, the scientific research that supports the use of pellets to replace estradiol and testosterone has been continuously published and documented since 1939. In fact, the use of pellets, like the type used in SottoPelle® Therapy, have been used in the United States since 1939 and can only be made in a compounding pharmacy. The amazing thing is how much this treatment modality has been ignored by the physician-training programs in the United States. Of course, research money is, in great part, supplied by pharmaceutical companies. What company wants stiff competition against the products it produces and promotes?

It seems that a solution this simple would be available to everyone, but the opposite is true. There are very few practitioners using this form of therapy. Why? Physicians are never exposed to this in specialty training because they are schooled only in the "traditional" forms of hormone therapy. The trend and desire for "natural" forms of hormone replacement has stimulated patients to look for physicians who employ not just natural but bio-identical hormones.

Chapter 6
Can SottoPelle® help with these?

There are some very serious health issues which plague individuals who, for one reason or another, have become hormonally deficient. As you will see, restoring your body back to its natural hormonal balance will help instill a greater sense of well-being and normalized body functions.

Menstrual Migraine

Dr. Somerville in the journal, Neurology, 1970 found that women who developed headaches prior to and during their menstrual periods responded favorably to estrogen therapy. To explore the viability and impact that estradiol pellets might make on menstrual migraines, I began treating women of all ages suffering with menstrual migraines with SottoPelle® estradiol pellets. In all cases, a small dose of pellet estradiol was inserted, and within three to seven days estrogen levels were elevated but more importantly, the estradiol levels were higher during the premenstrual and menstrual period and the patients' headaches were reduced significantly or eliminated. I have treated women from 22 to 49 years of age with menstrual migraines with over 90% success in eliminating their headaches. For anyone who is incapacitated with this form of migraine headache, SottoPelle® estradiol can be a godsend.

Ovarian Cancer

This cancer is a type of female cancer that is, unfortunately, most commonly diagnosed in its advanced stages. Early-stage tumors are most commonly not found, which is when they are most treatable and curable.

How then can the use of SottoPelle® Therapy impact ovarian cancer? The most compelling argument is found in the research that demonstrates birth control pills effectively reduce the incidence of ovarian cancer by up to 70%. This is the only effective way ovarian cancer can be "treated." Prevent it. The question arises, how do birth control pills effect this beneficial result? The answer I believe lies in the extremely low levels of FSH (follicle stimulating hormone) that birth control pills produce which keep the ovaries quiet and inactive. With this information taken into account, the primary goal for physicians should be to keep the FSH level in *postmenopausal* women as low as the levels produced by birth control pills. The hormones in birth control pills are synthetic, and the only biologically-identical estradiol that suppresses the FSH continually and as effectively as birth control pills is found in estradiol pellets. Oral forms and creams do not suppress the FSH. (Elevated levels of FSH continually bombard the ovary with stimulation. Decreasing stimulation by FSH reduces the occurrence of ovarian cancer). During the ten-year period from 1992 to 2002, there have been no documented cases of ovarian cancer among the more than 1,000 patients I have treated with SottoPelle® Therapy. All of these patients have very low FSH levels. To summarize, if you don't allow the ovary to be stimulated, you reduce the chance of ovarian cancer. The only form of bio-identical hormone that accomplishes this is estradiol SottoPelle® Therapy.

Post Partum Depression

This devastating disease that develops shortly after the wondrous miracle called birth goes untreated frequently and can have disastrous results for mother, baby, and the whole family. How does this develop? The obvious answer is that the body, just after the placenta is removed, is robbed of all of its hormone (estradiol, progesterone and testosterone) production. Therefore, the goal would be to effectively elevate the hormone levels with bio-identical estradiol. The use of bio-identical hormones given in SottoPelle® Therapy poses no threat to infants that are breast-feeding. If it did, then breastfed babies of mothers who have started menstruating again would have problems because menstruating breast feeding mothers are producing all their hormones. The only form of therapy that can do this safely is SottoPelle® Therapy, because of the extremely low levels of hormones utilized. Furthermore, this hormone is absorbed directly into the bloodstream and the liver is bypassed, making it safe for mother and child. The best part is it starts to work in 36-72 hours. Think of the number of women whose post-partum suffering could be eliminated. This therapy does not interfere with antidepressant medications.

Osteoporosis

The oldest therapy for the elimination of osteoporosis is estrogen replacement therapy. There are as many deaths from complications of osteoporosis as there are from breast cancer (50,000 per year). This disease needs to be treated aggressively, and synthetic hormone therapy should be avoided. In 1990, J.W.W. Studd, M.D., demonstrated that oral estrogen increases bone density only 1 – 2% and patch estrogen 3.5%, but estradiol pellets elevated bone density 8.3% annually.

"...oral oestregen [estrogen] in general increases vertebral bone density by approximately 1-2% per annum (Linsay, et al, 1976; Christiansen and Christiansen, 1981), whereas the 75mg oestradiol [estradiol] implant, which achieves oestradiol [estradiol] levels in general at least double those of oral therapy, has been shown to increase vertebral bone density by 8.3% per annum" (Smith/Studd, British Journal of Hospital Medicine, 1993).

If a therapy is to be used, it should be safe and easily tolerated. No safer estrogen is available than bio-identical estradiol, and SottoPelle® Therapy is the best way to deliver it to the bone. Estradiol SottoPelle® Therapy is absorbed directly into the bloodstream and none is lost. No other form of providing estrogen to the body can deliver such doses at continual, steady levels, which is necessary for optimum bone growth. This is why estradiol pellets have been an important mode of therapy for osteoporosis in the United Kingdom since 1990. In fact my wife who developed osteoporosis at 43 years of age, was found to have normal bone density after one year of SottoPelle® hormone therapy without any other medications.

Vaginal Atrophy

A very frequent complaint from women is vaginal dryness which causes pain with intercourse. The atrophy (thinning) of the vaginal lining, and loss of muscle tone from the lack of estrogen and testosterone in postmenopausal women may produce profound physical and emotional problems for them, and their significant others. The thinning of the vagina causes dryness, loss of lubrication, and pain with intercourse from the trauma produced by excess friction. The loss of muscle tone accelerates the development of uterine and vaginal prolapse. Prolapse is defined as loss of support for the uterus, bladder, and rectum. This prolapse frequently leads to surgery to correct the problems that accompany its development (urinary and rectal incontinence, excess pelvic pressure). The use of SottoPelle® estradiol and testosterone therapy treats both of the problems safely. The estradiol thickens the vagina, and the combination of estradiol and testosterone allows the muscles to thicken and tone. The use of SottoPelle® Therapy together with proper exercise can help to avoid surgery.

Chronic Fatigue Syndrome and Fibromyalgia

Many patients are affected by these diseases. I often find elevated levels of antibodies to the Epstein-Barr virus which causes mononucleosis in adolescents and chronic fatigue in adults. I also often find low testosterone levels in both chronic fatigue and Fibromyalgia and have used SottoPelle® Therapy testosterone pellets to correct the hormone deficiencies, resulting in increased energy and a better quality of life. The traditional therapies used for both need to be continued, but adding testosterone helps these patients regain a better quality of life.

Patients with HIV or AIDS

Those affected by these diseases often complain of fatigue and lethargy. Many HIV-positive men are being treated with synthetic testosterone to give them increased energy. Why utilize synthetic testosterone when biologically identical testosterone is available? With so many drugs utilized in the treatment of HIV and AIDS, the liver needs to be protected. Synthetic testosterone does not afford this protection, but testosterone pellets do give this protection. My male patients feel stronger and have a better quality of life and better physical strength.

Breast Cancer

The development of breast cancer with the use of oral conjugated estrogens and synthetic progesterone was found to increase breast cancer after ten years. (WIH study). But in fact biologically identical hormone could be breast protective. The best form of biologically identical hormone that gives normal levels of estradiol to the breast tissue is SottoPelle® estradiol pellets. In a study I just completed, 967 women were studied from 1992 till 2002. In this group of women using SottoPelle® Therapy, there has been only **one** case of breast cancer. 40% of this group of women were taking biologically identical progesterone as well. Theoretically in this ten-year period, there should have been over 100 cases of breast cancer, because the incidence of breast cancer in women of all ages is one out of nine.

Therefore, if one out of nine women will get breast cancer whether they are taking or not taking hormones, you would think that over 100 of my patients would have developed breast cancer. Why didn't this happen? Estradiol pellets release a tiny amount of hormone daily. It releases only a biologically identical hormone, and does not produce excess stimulation of the estrogen receptors in the breast. From looking at the above numbers, you could easily say that the form of estrogen replacement therapy might be breast protective.

Another consideration is the patient who has had breast cancer. What can be done to improve her quality of life? Too often these patients suffer with severe hot flashes, loss of libido, mood swings and generally not feeling like their old self. The use of SottoPelle® testosterone therapy to improve their problem has been very successful. Dr. D. Gambrill who has been using estrogen and testosterone pellets to treat breast cancer patients recently published the safety of this therapy with excellent results, and has less cancer reoccurrence than patients not using pellet hormones.

Chapter 7
I feel alive again!

In light of all that has been said, it is important to create a new list, a list of how great you should feel with a properly balanced hormonal system. After having taken so many pills for so long, it may seem almost impossible that just a few, rice-sized pellets, like the type used in SottoPelle® Therapy, can actually provide all that your body needs. Because they are not ingested into your stomach, then processed by your liver, many of the flavorings, buffers, and excess "medicines" are not required. When your body is low in either estrogen or testosterone, it seeks a source, finds what it needs from the pellets, and processes and utilizes it immediately. Because of this, people using SottoPelle® Therapy:

- Feel much more in control of their bodies and their lives

- Sleep more consistently and soundly

- Are more interested in sex
- Realize greater mental clarity
- Enjoy renewed vitality and zest
- Are more enthusiastic
- Are calm, relaxed and stable
- Achieve better results with exercise (less effort more results)
- Secure additional benefits like increasing their bone mass (as much as 4 times greater than oral hormones) experience reduced menstrual migraines, and reduce their fears about breast cancer because SottoPelle® Therapy does not stimulate breast tissue.

The only form of therapy that satisfies the body's hormonal need are subcutaneous (under the skin) SottoPelle® estradiol and testosterone therapy. Lets review what we covered about SottoPelle® Therapy:

- Are they biologically identical? Yes!

The hormones are derived from soy, and more importantly hand- compounded to be the biologically identical human form of estradiol and testosterone. The body has what it can no longer produce.

• Is it effective and hassle free? Yes!

SottoPelle® is the only form of hormone therapy that effectively reduces to normal levels the body's FSH (follicle stimulating hormone). The elevation of FSH in women and men causes anxiety, irritability, hot flashes, lethargy and loss of well-being. The other forms of therapy require high doses of hormones to affect this. Pellet hormone therapy requires minute amounts of hormones to effect this lowering of FSH.

• Are they biologically available? Yes!

The pellets, once implanted, work automatically. The hormones are secreted in tiny amounts daily and when more hormone is needed (i.e. stress and exercise) the body will receive more hormone. This is caused by the rise of the heart rate causing increased blood flow over the pellets and in the case of exercise increased thermal release from muscles being exercised. <u>No other form of hormone administration can do this</u>.

<u>SottoPelle® Therapy is hassle-free</u> and can last for four to six months. The quality of life that is given back to patients utilizing SottoPelle® Therapy is second to none. I

know this because I hear it many times a day and use SottoPelle® testosterone therapy myself.

• Is it safe? Yes!

SottoPelle® Therapy hormones are biologically identical and absorbed directly. Therefore, no liver involvement is necessary. The hormones also don't interfere with medications for heart disease, high blood pressure, kidney disease, or thyroid disease. Biologically identical hormone does not increase the risk of breast cancer.

The only difference between SottoPelle® Therapy for men compared to women is the amount of hormones needed. Men consume more testosterone than women consume estrogen and testosterone. The amount of time between treatments is the same, the procedure is the same, and most importantly, the overall positive results are the same. With SottoPelle® Therapy, men will realize:

• Restored sexual drive

• Relief from hormone-related depression

• Consistency—no more roller coaster effect compared to oral therapies, injections, creams or gels

- Elevated energy levels
- Greater capacity for getting in shape
- Increased mental clarity and focus
- Decreased body fat
- Improved erectile ability
- Improved mental clarity, focus and concentration

Here are just a few of the hundreds of testimonials I have received from patients who have regained their hormonal vigor through SottoPelle® Therapy.

"I tried it all, Premarin, patches, creams-you name it! No matter what I used, I still felt just as bad. After SottoPelle® Therapy, my life began!"

- Mrs. Patty from California

"Thank you for changing my life. At age 38 I am feeling like 18 again and a lot happier."

- Mrs. Elmira from California

"I had a hysterectomy six years ago. My friend said I had been scaring her with my mood swings and instability. Now I'm me again! My husband even says he can see the young woman he married 20 years ago."

- Mrs. Deborah from California

"For the first time since my hysterectomy in 1989, I actually feel so wonderful. I felt bad for so long I forgot what it was like to have lots of energy, no leg cramps, no night sweats, able to think straight, able to sleep all night, and to have sexual desires again. I am a new woman!"

- Mrs. Patty from California

"After working 13 hours on Monday and 14 hours on Tuesday from being a floor nurse, I got home last night and I wanted sex out of the blue. My husband was expecting a cranky worn out nurse and got a 35-ish wow- mamma. I feel 35."

- Mrs. Judi from Kansas

"For five years I have tried every combination of hormone replacement therapy to treat my symptoms, to no avail. With each passing year my symptoms of night sweats, huge temperature shifts, sleeplessness and depression were getting worse. I found that menopause was definitely not for sissies! I was anxious to try anything. With the SottoPelle® Therapy, I couldn't have hoped for a better outcome. Within two weeks I was sleeping through the night with NO night sweats. My tempera-

ture comfort zone has normalized. I can't describe what a difference it has made in my quality of life. I would recommend SottoPelle® Therapy to anyone who is ready to live life normally again!"

- Ms. Carol from California

"I just wanted to let you know how much better I felt almost immediately after I had my first SottoPelle® Therapy treatment. I actually felt peppier, I have slept better, been much more patient, and had much more energy. I also used to have head-aches almost every day, many times all day long. But now I find I hardly ever take any pain medication for them. My hormone levels were much improved after three weeks. I look forward to feeling this good for a long time."

- Mrs. Eileen from California

"For five years, I took testosterone shots and used adhesive patches. Because I am an active person, the patches did not stick, and besides, they just didn't give me enough help to make them worth the has-sle. The shots made my hemoglobin shoot way up. That is not what I wanted. What I really wanted was something that was *a lot more permanent, less bothersome, and more effective. My daughter told me that I should try SottoPelle® Therapy. Since I started SottoPelle® Therapy, I am my old self again! My wife is delighted that I have regained my former "zip" that had been missing for so long."*

- Mr. Robert from Missouri

I am a husband, father, athlete, entrepreneur, volunteer but, during the past couple of years my physical and mental energy and sexual desire began to dramatically fall off. My wife was a patient of Dr. Tutera's and she was raving about her positive results with the SottoPelle® treatment. I was too! She convinced me... and the results have been beyond our expectations! I encourage all men who feel the way I did to contact the people at SottoPelle®...You'll feel better about yourself and so will everyone around you.

- Mr. Jim from California

Conclusion
I'm ready to begin!

After you have completed your reading of all the previous pages, you should know far more about how your body works, what to ask for concerning proper diagnostic tests and how to distinguish bio-identical from bio-equivalent HRT options. You should also understand the powerful and dynamic benefits SottoPelle® Therapy provides.

Bio-identical hormones are the only choice for helping to reinvigorate your life without the nasty side effects of the more traditional HRT treatment options. Your body wants what it originally was designed to have. Bio-identical, natural, subcutaneous pellet therapy is the only HRT option that will reestablish a normal hormonal process in your body.

SottoPelle® Therapy will enable you to enjoy:

• A restored sexual drive

- Relief from hormone-related depression

- Consistency! No more roller coaster effect compared to oral therapies and/or injections

- Elevated energy levels

- Greater capacity for getting in shape

- Increased mental clarity and focus

- Substantially diminished fears and frustrations concerning traditional HRT

The only form of hormone therapy that is truly effective, without problematic side-effects, is SottoPelle® Therapy. I am dedicated to making this form of therapy available to every woman and man for replacement of those precious hormones that benefit, protect, and energize our lives.

Pellet hormone therapy has been utilized in the United States since 1939 but has never caught on because of the popularity of synthetic compounds and horse hormone. **It's time for a change.**

If you are like most patients I see, you are probably anxious to find a physician who can help you with SottoPelle® Therapy. Visit our website at www.sottopelletherapy.com to find a trained physician near you. Or perhaps your physician may be interested in contacting me about adopting SottoPelle® Therapy. There is a growing list of physicians who are using SottoPelle® Therapy who have also been trained by me in the full and complete processes of diagnosis and extensive monitoring of this type of therapy. Instead of listing them here, I suggest that you go to my website for more complete information. We are always updating it so that it will serve as a viable resource for you at all times. Please visit:

www.sottopelletherapy.com

I have enjoyed sharing my insights and experience with you over the course of these pages. **Whatever you do, please remember that a healthy, well-balanced and exciting life can once again be yours.**

1. Salmon U., et al.: Use of estradiol subcutaneous pellets in humans. Science 1939,90:162.

2. Mishel, D.: Clinical study of estrogenic therapy with pellet implantation. Am J Obstet-Gynecol 1941:41:1009.

3. Greenblatt, R.: Indications for hormone pellets in the therapy of endocrine and gynaecological disorders. American J Obstet Gyn, 1949:57:294.

4. Studd, J.: Estradiol and testosterone implants in the treatment of psychosexual problems in postmenopausal women. Br. J Obstet Gynaecol 1977:84:314.

5. Thom, M., Studd, J., Oestorgen/testosterone implant therapy. In: Oestrogens and the Menopause. Edited by M. I. Whitehead & J. W. W. Studd. Abbott Labs, London, 1978: 85

6. "Oral preparations, unlike implants, also reduce liver metabolism of clotting factors and lipids" Elkik F., Gompel A., MTP Press 103-25

7. Lobo, R.: Subdermal estradiol pellets following hysterectomy and oophorectomy. Am J Obstet Gynecol 1980:138:714.

8. Thom, M., et al.: Hormone implantation. Br. Med J 1980:1:848.

9. Thom, M., et al.: Hormone profiles in postmenopausal women after therapy with subcutaneous implants. Br J Obstet Gynaecol 1981:88:426.

10. Brincat, M., et al.: Subcutaneous hormone implants for the control of climacteric symptoms. Lancet 1984:1:16.

11. Burger, H., et al.: The management of persistent menopausal symptoms with oestradiol-testosterone implants: clinical, lipid and hormone results. Maturitas 1984:6:351.

12. Cardoza, L., et al.: The effects of subcutaneous hormone implants during climacteric. Maturitas 1984:5:177.

13. Farish, E., et al.: The effects of hormone implants on serum lipoproteins and steroid hormones in bilaterally oophorectomised women. Acta Endocrinol (Copenh) 1984:106:116.

14. Barlow, D., et al.: Long-term hormone implants therapy-hormonal and clinical effects. Obstet & Gynecol 1986:67:321.

15. Burger, H., et al.: Effect of combined implants of oestradiol and testosterone on libido in postmenopausal women. Br Med J 1987:294:936.

16. Notelovitz, M., et al.: Metabolic and hormonal effects of 50 mgm 17 B Estradiol Implants in surgically menopausal women. Obstet-Gynecol 1987:70:749.

17. Greenblatt, R., et al.: Indications for hormonal pellets in the therapy of gynecologic disorders. Am J Obstet-Gynecol 1988:159:1540.

18. Savvas, M., et al.: Skeletal effects of oral oestrogen compared with subcutaneous oestrogen and

testosterone in postmenopausal women. Br Med J 1988:279:331.

19. Stanczyk, F., et al.: A randomized comparison of nonoral estradiol delivery in postmenopausal women. Am J Obstet Gynecol 1988:159:1540.

20. Studd, J., et al.: The relationship between plasma estradiol and the increase in bone density in postmenopausal women after treatment with subcutaneous hormone implants. Am J Obstet Gynecol 1990:63:1474.

21. Savvas, M., et al.: Increase in bone mass after one year of percutaneous oestradiol and testosterone implants in postmenopausal women who have previously received oral oestrogens. Br J Obstet Gynaecol 1992:99:757.

22. Smith, RNJ; Studd, J.W.W. Recent Advances in Hormone Replacement Therapy, British Journal of Hospital Medicine 1993.

23. Holland, E., et al.: The effect of 25-mg percutaneous estradiol implants on the bone mass of postmenopausal women. Obstet Gynecol 1994:83:43.

24. Davis, S., et al.: Testosterone enhances estradiol's effects on postmenopausal bone density and sexuality. Maturitas 1995:21:227.

25. Handelsman, D., Androgen Delivery Systems: Testosterone Pellet Implants: Pharma Bio: 1986: 459:467.

26. Natrajan, P., et al.: Estrogen replacement therapy in women with previous breast cancer: Presented at

the Sixty-first Annual Meeting of The South Atlantic Association of Ob/Gyn, White Sulfur Springs, West Va, Jan. 23-26: 1999.

27. Davis, S., et al.: Effects of estradiol with and without testosterone on body composition and relationships with lipids in postmenopausal women. Menopause: The J No Am Meno Soc 2000: 395.

28. Sands RH, S., et al. The effect of hormone replacement therapy and route of administration on selected cardiovascular risk factors in post-menopausal women. Fam Pra GB: 2000 Vol. 17, No. 6.

29. Cravioto, M., et al.: Pharmacokenietics and Pharmacodynamics of 25-mg estroadiol implants in postmenopausal Mexican women. The J No Am Meno Soc 2001: Vol. 8. No. 5: 353:360.

30. Pirwany, I., et al.: Supraphysiological concentrations of estradiol in menopausal women given repeated implant therapy do not adversely affect lipid profiles. European Soc Hum Rep Emb 2002: Vol.17,No.3 pp. 825:829.

GINO TUTERA, M.D., F.A.C.O.G.

Currently, Medical Director of SottoPelle® — A Center for Hormonal Balance & Well-Being, Scottsdale, AZ and Palm Desert, CA

Licensure
- State of Missouri, 1971
- State of California, 1993
- State of Arizona, 2000

Medical Director of OB/GYN at Baptist Medical Center, Kansas City, MO, 1981-1984

Medical Director of Kansas City PMS Clinic, 1982-1992

Medical Director, Women's Center at Baptist Medical Center, Kansas City, MO, 1982— Created center dealing with women's health issues including education and reference library

Clinical Instructor for Obstetrics & Gynecology, Goppert Family Practice Residency, 1984-1987

Medical Director of the Hanson Birthing Center, Obstetrical Unit at Eisenhower Medical Center, Rancho Mirage, CA, 1992-1995

Chairman, Section of OB/GYN at Eisenhower Medical Center, Rancho Mirage, CA, 1996-1998

Vice Chairman, Department of Obstetrics & Gynecology, Baptist Medical Center, Kansas City, MO, 1989-1991

Diplomat of American Board of Obstetrics & Gynecology, 1977-Present

Fellow American College of Obstetrics & Gynecology, 1977-Present

Medical Society Memberships

Diplomat American Board of Obstetrics & Gynecology

Fellow American College of Obstetrics & Gynecology

American Medical Association

California Medical Association

Missouri Medical Association

American Association of Gynecologic Laparoscopists

American Society of Colposcopy and Cervical Pathology

A

Androgens - hormones that have male hormone effects in the human body (i.e. DHEA, Testosterone, etc.)

Arrhythmia - irregular heart rate pattern.

Aromatase - an enzyme in the human body that causes testosterone (a male hormone) to be changed to estrogen (female hormone) and vice versa.

ACTH - a hormone from a gland in the brain called the pituitary. It regulates the adrenal glands in the body.

Addison's Disease - a disease of the adrenal glands. This life threatening disease results from the adrenal glands being unable to produce cortisol; the body's cortisone.

Atrophy - loss of tissue thickness.

Androstenedione - (An-dro-steen-dye-own) a hormone that has weaker male effects than testosterone. Often seen as a supplement called "Andro." Actually a hormone the body makes which is then transformed into testosterone and even estrogen.

Augment - to enlarge or to intensify an effect.

Andropause - "Male Menopause." The male body is no longer able to produce enough testosterone.

B

Bio-equivalent - a term meaning a substance has effects similar to the biologic substance it's replacing, but does not have the exact chemical structure.

Bio-identical - a substance is identical to the substance it is replacing in both effect and chemical structure.

C

Cholesterol - a fat in the blood.

HDL - the good cholesterol.

LDL & VLDL - bad cholesterol.

Cortex - the outer shell of a body organ or gland.

Cushing's syndrome - a disease of the adrenal glands that causes the glands to over produce cortisol, causing high blood pressure, marked weight gain, muscle wasting, fluid retention, and loss of bone density.

D

Diabetes - a disease caused by the pancreas not being able to produce enough insulin hormone so that the body can use sugars properly.

DHEA - a weak male hormone produced by the body which is then changed into testosterone.

E

Endocrine System - the body has a group of glands that secrete their hormones directly into the blood stream and are called the endocrine system i.e.: the thyroid, pituitary, etc.

Endocrinology - the study of the endocrine glands and their function.

Enzyme - a protein in the body that is used to start, speed up, or eliminate a particular chemical reaction in the body.

Epinephrine - the other name for the body's "Adrenaline."

Equilin - the primary estrogen hormone in horses. The primary hormone in the drugs: Premarin™, Prempro™, and Premphase.™

Estradiol - the primary female hormone of the human body. The workhorse estrogen for human females.

Estrogen - female hormones.

Estrone - one of the human female hormones, a very strong breast stimulator.

Estriol - a very weak estrogen made from estrone.

F

FSH - Follicle Stimulating Hormone, the hormone made by the pituitary that regulates the female ovary and male testicle. It regulates the hormone production of these organs.

Feedback Mechanism - the system in the human body which regulates the creation and release of hormones from the endocrine glands.

First Pass - First Pass Metabolism is the process in which the liver processes medicines in the liver cells.

Follicle cells - cells in the ovary that produce estrogen.

Follicular cells - cells in the thyroid gland that produce thyroid hormone.

G

Greenblatt, Robert, M. D. - one of the first physicians in America to use hormone pellets. First published his research in 1949.

I

Insulin - the hormone produced by the pancreas (an endocrine gland) that regulates the body's blood sugar. A deficiency of insulin causes the disease diabetes.

Islets of Langerhans - the cells in the pancreas that produce insulin.

L

LH - Leutenizing hormone (loo-teen-eye-zing). The pituitary hormone that controls ovulation and progesterone hormone production in a woman, and testosterone in a man.

M

Medulla - a term that refers to the middle of an organ or gland.

Menopause - the time of life when a women stops ovulating, and stops producing enough estrogen, the female hormone.

Menstrual Migraine - a severe headache that comes only around the time of a women's menstrual period. Probably caused by low estrogen levels.

N

Norepinephrine - the other adrenaline the adrenal glands produce.

O

Osteopenia - decreased bone density sufficient enough to increase the fracture risk in human bones.

Osteoporosis - severe bone density loss which results in a very high fracture risk.

Ovary - the female reproductive endocrine organ. The ovaries are positioned one on each side of the uterus.

Ovulation - the process of expelling the female egg from the ovary.

P

Pancreas - the endocrine organ that is located in the belly that produces digestive enzymes, and the hormone insulin.

Progesterone - the hormone produced from the ovary after the egg has been expelled. Usually only produced in significant amounts for 10-12 days of each menstrual cycle. High levels are only seen in pregnancy.

Pregnenalone - a hormone made from progesterone which the body creates on the way to making estrogen and testosterone.

Prolactin - the hormone produced by the back portion of the pituitary gland (posterior pituitary) which causes milk production and milk let down from the female breast.

Prolapse - a term used to indicate a loss of support for the uterus, (i.e.: uterine prolapse) which caused the uterus to drop lower into the vagina.

Pulmonary embolus - a usually fatal condition caused by a blood clot being released (thrown) to the lung, commonly from the leg veins or pelvic veins.

R

Rectal incontinence - the loss of control of the anal sphincter muscle which causes fecal material to exit.

"Roller Coaster Effect" - the up and down of hormone levels produced by pills, patches, creams and shots. This does not occur with hormone pellet usuage.

S

Salivary glands - glands in the mouth that produce saliva (spit) and deliver it through a tiny tube called a duct.

SHBG - sex hormone binding globulin – a protein which can attach itself to estrogen or testosterone and make them unavailable for the body to absorb from the blood.

Sheehan's Syndrome - results from a partial or complete loss of blood supply to the pituitary gland. This results in partial or complete loss of the pituitary's ability to produce its hormones, and can lead to the loss of thyroid hormone, estrogen hormone production, testosterone production, and adrenal gland function which could result in serious illness or death if not properly treated.

Subcutaneous - "under the skin", the fatty layer that lies just under the skin.

T

Testicle - the male sex gland;. It produces sperm and testosterone hormones.

Testosterone - the male hormone; an androgen.

TSH - thyroid stimulating hormone. The hormone produced by the pituitary gland that controls the creation and release of the two thyroid hormones.

T3 - triodothyronine (try-eye-odo-thigh-row-neen) - one of two thyroid hormone.

T4 - thyroxine (thigh-rock-sin) – one of two thyroid hormone.

U

Urinary Incontinence - the inability to control the loss of urine from the bladder.

V

Vaginal Atrophy - the loss of the normal lining and the thickness of the vagina which makes a women feel dry and causes discomfort during sexual intercourse.